The Shoulders of Country Roads

My Journey from Head and Neck Cancer

The Shoulders of Country Roads

My Journey from Head and Neck Cancer

Susan Singer Kerschner

Parisburg Publishing

Photography by author except as noted.
Book design: Author
Cover photograph: T. Weihe
Inset photo back cover: Reagan Singer
Author photographs: W. Dolen

First Edition
Third Printing

Copies available:
www.amazon.com
www.barnesandnoble.com

ISBN-13: 978-1-619180-10-9
1. Poetry. 2. Cancer.

Parisburg Publishing
www.parisburg.com

for those traveling this road

LIFELONG THANKS

This compilation of poems is in memory of Joseph Treceno, beat poet and artiste extraordinaire, who believed in me as an authentic poet and persuaded me to write this book. Bless your darling spirit, Joe.

For my precious parents, Patricia Main and Arnold Singer, for their absolute love and care; my sister Lisa Kelly who repeatedly flew across country; my brother Reagan Singer who rapidly arranged for airline tickets and the best doctors in the country; my nephew and niece, Grayson and Paige, who lovingly monitored my boo-boo and made me laugh every single day.

To my cousin Lorrie Singer, her husband Bradley Kopp and my beloved, recently departed sister Debbie Mohney Hoyes who often traveled the road from Austin; my sister Jacqueline Singer, niece Elise Kelly, cousins, friends for their sustaining cards, texts, calls, visits and emails; David Webb for his song-a-day; extended family Elizabeth Young and Cynthia Russ who provided tender care, special gifts, airfare when I needed it most.

Gratefully to Dawn and Chris Thren, my guardian angels, and Phyllis Singer my devoted stepmother, who timelessly carted me around MD Anderson explaining the cancer center ropes, sharing her own daring excursions to and from the world of cancer.

Blessings to Cather and Russ for their exquisite friendship, doctor and airport runs and the soothing comforts of home. Special acknowledgment to Mary Twyman, RN who called daily and spoke when I could not; and David Syer for the beautiful healing prayer quilt.

My brilliant doctors — Randal Weber, David Rosenthal, and Rony Dev, and the wonderful caretakers at MD Anderson whose intention was that I not suffer, despite universal fears about morphine addiction.

Most of all, greatest appreciation to my sister-in-law Carla Singer, who rearranged her life's routines to be at the critical center of my care.

To Life.

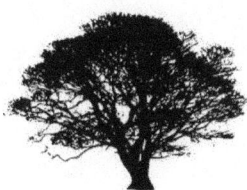

Contents

My Journey
from Head and Neck Cancer

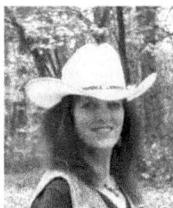

Fx

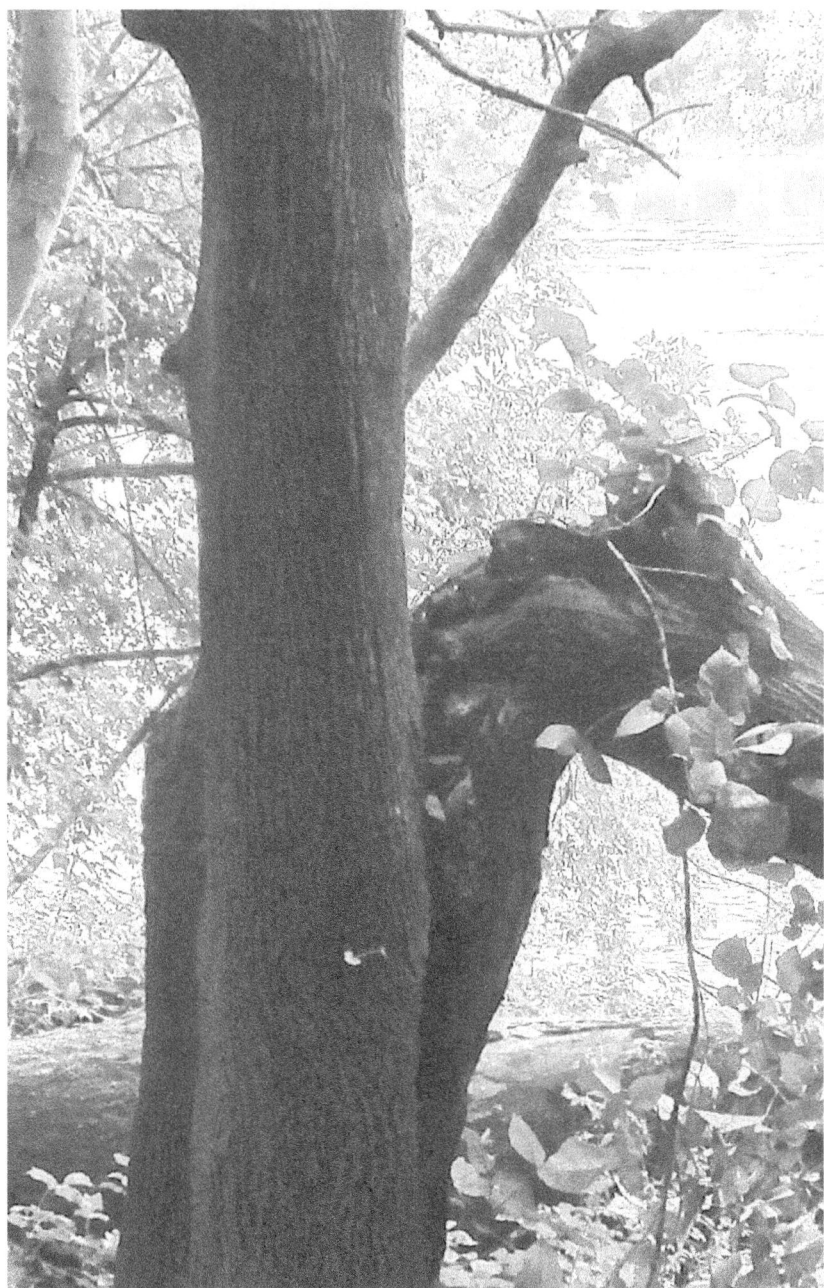

Fracture

Monument of marble and ash
attracts tourist eyes
once rolled upwards
in monolithic awe
now bent down
into pools of underground abyss
crevice, shatter, chasm, rupture

four friends on city sojourn
seated at local fare
conversation takes second violin
all eyes fixed on
curbside ice cream truck
restaurant pales in temptation
cranny, fault, flaw, splinter

in her more lucid days
family matriarch divvies up jewelry
granddaughters attend to gilded box
brimming with interlaced stories
sum of her life in objects
rift, gap, breach, flaw

midwestern town
appears unscathed
after tornado rips vegetation
eldest tree upended
rotund crater of calm destruction
fissure, gash, tear, cleft

something happens
to set the thing apart
from itself, from you
from everyone
it changes the story
slit, rent, break, opening

on the radio a song
Leonard Cohen instructs
there's a crack in everything
that's how the light gets in.

Dx

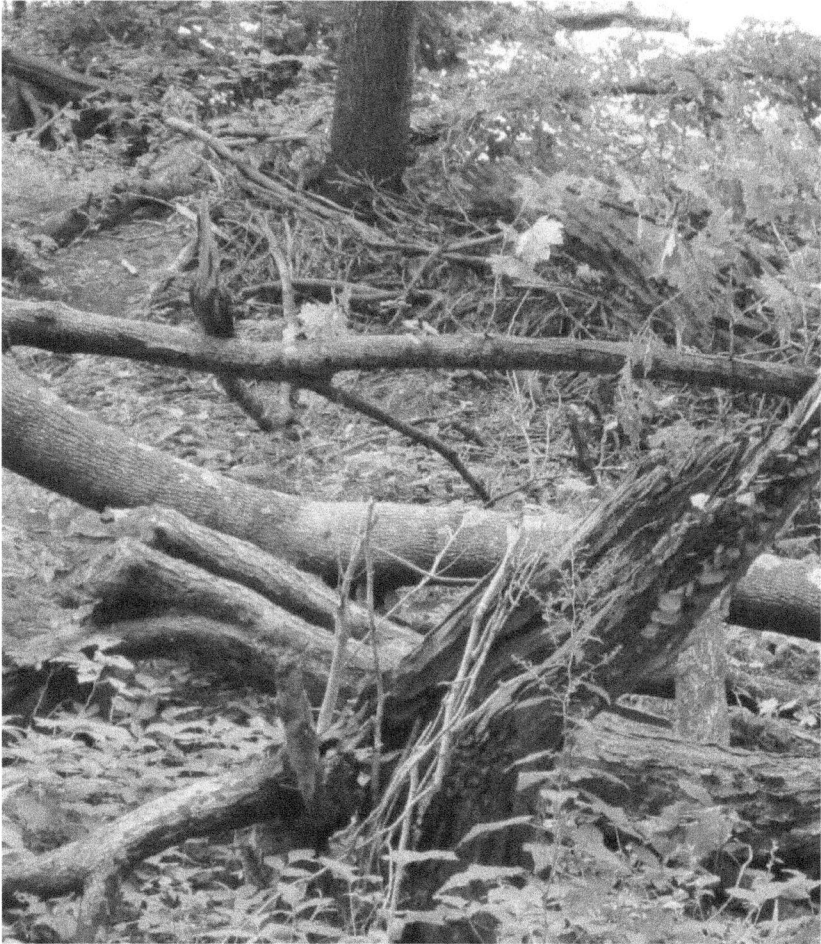

Mistake

Impatient doctor sends patient home
with metastatic lump in neck
that'll be a $30 co-pay
tells her *come back in a few weeks*

summer spent
in radiation sandwich
sending a thousand brown curls
from a burning pyre
scattering into autumn skies

husband lover
keeps his distance
fearful of what she will look like
what's so great about
transcendental sex anyway?

treatment sets fire to
speech
sound
aroma
taste
joy
in the name
of
healing

prostate and breast survivors
try to soothe
everyone goes through this
but do they breathe or eat
with penis or bosom?

with all its cognition
head doesn't warn
about consequences

it was a mistake
someone made

too much saccharine
monosodium glutamate
pesticide
microwave
food mutation
too much car exhaust
arsenic in wine grapes
cigarette smoke spewing
from collective lungs

it's a mistake
we're in this together

Bomb Shelter

With no warning
primary school air raid drills begin
deafening and shrill, unrelenting
siren files children into halls

crouched on shiny linoleum
hands behind necks
rows of lacy ankle socks
obscure classroom doorways

disembodied voice announcement
put your head between your knees
and NO talking

no one notices teachers
left standing
(safety is relative)
no child dares lift a head
threat of death looming
they wait for nothing to happen.

Shot full of mysterious fluids
cushioned table transports me
into a tunnel
medical technicians disappear

into safe room. No siren except
unembodied voice:
be still and don't swallow.

War is on: tracer armies
signal back to home base

planned places to attack
drills don't count here
this is *it*
machine clicks sounds
records images
plain socks warm my toes
silent prayer bears down

I am the ailing country
the Cuban target
crouching for safety
waiting for something to happen.

City of Isotopes

Satellite view
population clusters
map of the world
in lights
prominently displayed
its sparkling grid
embedded into a dark planet
look there to the left
Los Angeles   New York   Paris

l u m i n o s i t y

towns powered to appear
dense from a distance
buildings, conduit, nuclear statues
pimpling the universe
can't be seen from space

waste, pollution, poverty
have no impression here
towns swell to compete
for notoriety and permanence

I am Earth in a laboratory
geographically appointed
longitudes and latitudes
lined up for alien sightings

insignificant atoms
lit with radioactive isotopes
cancer cells congregate
with sugar-filled urgency

lightness

I dream I am clear
safe, not punctured with electricity
wanting to be a non-destination
not a milieu for molecules

just a city that wakes up bustling
without memory of night's
hidden colors or gamma rays
tracking unwanted strangers.

Foreign Body

Foreign
suggests bodily objects
that don't belong
plaguing cells
conflicting life messages
or angular
dancing Middle Eastern arms
perched on a pulpit
in continuous motion
incense and worship
conjure up indigenous struggle
leaders hope or pretend to abridge;
begun in the embryo of ancient days,
remote towns become familiar
military cells filled with soldiers.

But back to that foreign body
lesion, legion
that comes to a neighborhood
of blood and corpuscle
at war to take out a life
breathe in something
so far outside of us,
we find ourselves singing
in foreign tongues.

Tenth Floor

A building is like the body
take the elevator
starting from the bottom

destination:
Head and Neck
the place a PET scan begins
at the knees
a body's ground floor

Elevator A
up, up, up

gather bits of yourself on the elevator
pause on Two, Three
doors open on Four: *Pain Management*
a woman and her liver get off
holding her middle

stopover on Eight: *Apheresis & Leukemia*
like removal of whole blood from a patient,
guts of the crowd exits

hear snippets of patients' lives
without knowing them
malignant tumors wait their turn

on Nine
bone, cartilage, tissue, muscle
every stop a corresponding body part
door closes again
this fits your attention span

travel further to top of body
homo sapiens, building erectus
the thinking zone
decisions will be made
mild, moderate, radical
to execute neck dissection

depart sooner than you expect
lifetimes divide
multiply in slow motion

wait for the *Ding*
where you're closest to resolution
the nth landing of wellness.

Haiku

Exploratory
slicing through unchartered land
uncovers blemish

Life or death conflict
who decides the time is now
or which flowers wilt

Big words are uttered
flood of vocabulary
relearn the simple

Volcanic future
nowhere to run for shelter
adverse elements

Tx

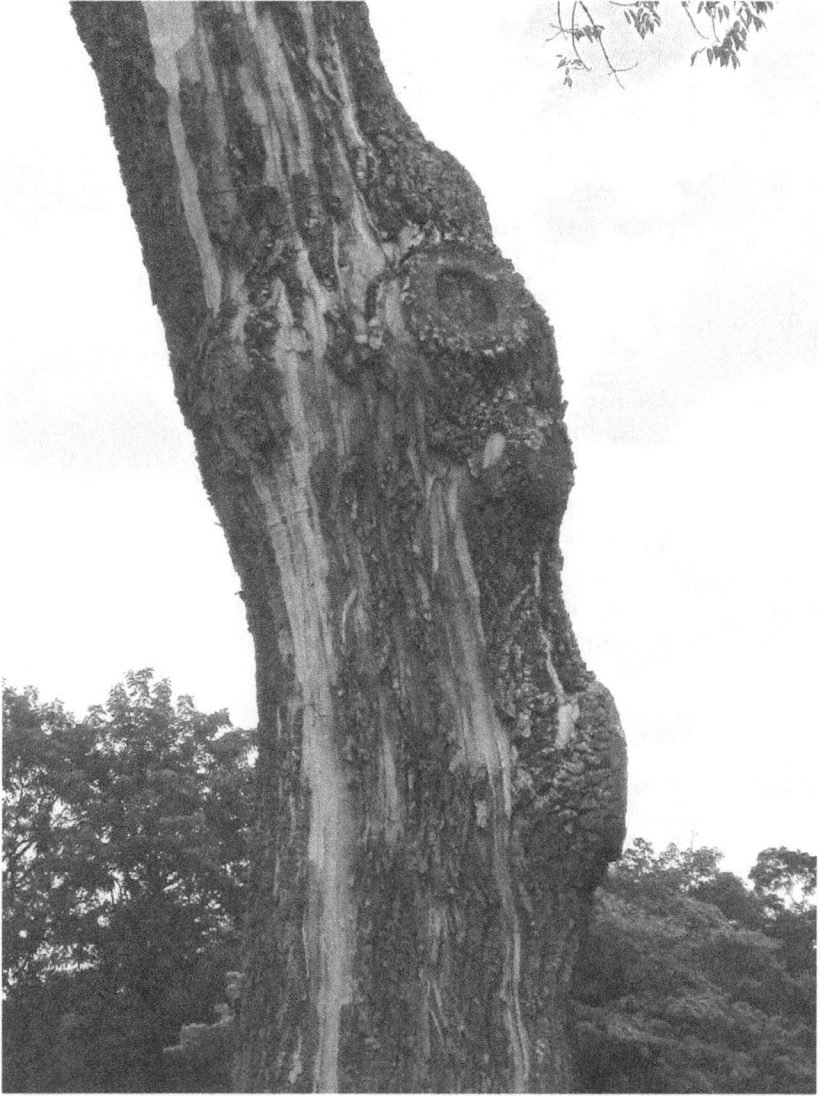

The Shoulders of Country Roads

Today my six-year old nephew asks
if Susu didn't go to her appointments
would she be dead?
It doesn't startle me
his tiny feather-soft hand inside mine
reassures me the sun is still
beaming incandescent angles of light
through the trees all around me
they welcome their own kind of healing

the ride to the Radiation Center
has its joys too
in his final ride to the guillotine
even the solipsist felt a keen awareness
of sharp colors
of deep lines around eyes of onlookers
of invisible angels shaking trees branches
hovering in the lowering sunset

dusk has a certain feel
on the side of a meandering lane
expired crispy leaves show renewed life
when they dance to a passing car
bending and twisting
nature rearranges, resettles herself
nothing ever stays the same

we can't recognize a curve
where we stopped to take a picture
of the convergence of hundreds
of white bark trunks
where an elk might have crossed earlier

the moments we pause to catch
our proverbial breath
have years between them
as the shoulders of country
roads stretch for miles.

Birth Rite

We were not zygotes splitting apart
but souls emerging
from the same fragile womb
sisters now endure the cancer eating my flesh
they cradle me with their goading
bossiness, desperation
challenge me on the playground
of our competitiveness
how dare you get sick?

They struggle to breathe
if they imagine the 'minus one'
the missing middle
inconceivable to be relieved
of three's a crowd
it's the taking for granted
that compels primeval devotion.

Driving in the hot Texas sun
closed car windows mask an illusory cool
the eldest speeds her sister
to some comfort of stark bed
fluorescent lamp
cold linoleum tomb;
needles and plastic await.

Highway offering of bumps and agony
pump up the music volume
a million apologies
we're almost there... almost there.

Little sister paces in distant coastal town
waiting for news, healing, anything
Roentgen rays that rescued the core
of my beginning, my middle, my unknown
and now invisible flames engulf a neck
ear, esophagus, nothing spared
artificial sun is slow to burn
boils, fries, sears to eruption.

Transference is not an option
like twins passing in and out
of each others' bodies and souls
but as mothers yearning to vanquish
pain from an aching child.

We are beyond interchangeable
like clothes that go back and forth for years
or *your doll looks better than mine*
now eyes/lungs/liver/skin shared.

Awake in the early hour
she lies on the gurney
with her sister's anguish
feeling the jerks
and blows to wounds
waits for time to pass.

A bond infiltrates beyond cell walls
she rushes from room-to-room change
memorizing the dip of her sibling's
head on a fresh pillow, to know

she'll be cared for
when the lights go out
and imagines a chromosomal lifting
the memory foam of our distant birthing.

On a Scale of Zero to Ten

Rate your pain.
Ten being I can't tolerate a second more
of this spontaneously burning forest
directly NNW of tired torso
body without soul
house on fire with a person inside
no room for philosophy or
discussion of recent eagle migration.

Shade trees are yanked from their base
just as invisible enemy removes skin
like a silent bulldozer
a kind of slash and burn
long after land is cleared
nutrient retooling
with a battle-specific scar.

Does earth feel a similar fibrosis,
its tall tottering banyons
facing physical displacement?
Stealth of forced tissue destruction
earns a rating of an Olympic competitor.
Let's hope for a five today.

Construction Zone

Serene sight through the bouquet-
topped window sill hides
the force of workers reconstructing
fire zones of radiation
and chemical warfare.

Hospital window angled just right
cranes poised for the morning bell
office cells rise in steel and concrete stages
adjacent hospital towers
house compromised capillaries
waiting for regeneration.

Never before has construction
looked so promising
while little men build like
ants from ground to sky.

Nurse, gauze needed in Room 53
Joe, move that beam to the right
weekend downtime
not a sound, just a bedside beep.
Which body will be rebuilt sooner?

Are skin and bone stronger
than ballast and girder?
Which will withstand
the tornado of illness?

Metaphor of the sick
riding the cranes
progress and life will resurrect
as bedridden eyes look out
a thousand double-paned windows.

At the Cellular Level

Something went wrong
refracted light
turn missed
broken sentence
body tries to correct itself
like low sun
throwing inescapable streaks
through a window
lying in wait
on the slab of morphine weariness
youth zapped by a thousand
invisible beams on a chrome board
not a bather on a beach
unsuspecting sun worship
prelude of raw skin
nights of sleepless agony ahead
world war metastasizes
silent injury
deep within
at the cellular level
tongue hurls a tidal wave of resistance
ear canal closes passage
no food or water
past this point
infantry poised for biological warfare
jaw recoils in defense
Arabian sandstorm of modern treatment
pronouns conspicuously missing
dictators toppled

a year stolen
a life regained
pronouns reappear
me
I
emerge.

Dignity

In a hospital bed
I lost my dignity
tall slender metallic
companion accompanies me
to the basin

we engage in momentary struggle
of who goes first. My free hand
repetitively douses my sole possession -
an off-the-shoulder, open-down-the-back
blue checked little number

grateful for the rectangular bar soap
I spare the nurses my embarrassment
thinking to myself how well I was raised
how much I want my mother

caregivers work hard to nurture me
to a better place. After fourteen
body scans, 32 neck scorchings
I become a handful

unable to make a sound
I watch the bustling
from inside a nimbus cloud
staying contained

I take in needles
cameras, fingers, rays
because they have to
break me down
to heal me

kill smooth skin
to grow new cells
burn out
to create rebirth
remove trees
to build a playground
starve the cancer
to save me

dignity is immaterial here
I scrub my gown
without feeling loss.

Simple Things

Hospital campus a half-country away
I am back in familiar surroundings
looking around I pretend
to do mindless chores
I pick up extraneous
belongings from each room,
placing clothes and objects
in some logical order.

I rest in a chair
normally unused
a formal Queen Anne
my mother gave me
situated to be admired
easy tasks have become hard
dust bunnies now in residence
bathroom porcelain begs to be shined
house accustomed to elbow grease
suffers in neglect.

The medical pronouncement
you are now free to go
to move about my life
turbulence has subsided
preparing me for the next six months
before poking and prodding restarts.
Brooms, mops, and pots await
mentally I do it all.

I lean back in the Queen Anne
to finish a dream
good cells accelerate

radiation is cleaning my house
it purges the cupboards of bad food
drinks properly-aged wine
exhausts itself
for me.

I remember under light sedation
my request to the surgeon
please don't disfigure me
as if he had a choice
10, 20 or 50 lymph nodes
things seem simple for everyone else
like broadcasting weather.

*Ok, today we have **two** sessions.*

That means the mask I wear
to immobilize me on the table
will be clamped to my head
against neck pus
at ten o'clock
again at four
pictures to be taken of my
ever-evolving cells
I imagine I am scrubbing floors.

It's CT Scan Monday, remember?

Meanwhile upstairs
through a waiting room window
a single sliver of sun cracks through
and damage from the previous day's
storm is forgotten.

Haiku

One more body scan
life on the horizontal
felled trees see life prone

Skin solar eclipse
pores erupt in rebellion
desert landscape torched

66 Gy Led the Big Parade

It takes brass
to submit to the force
of 66 Gy milligray photon radiation
make sure you pound the quarter notes
off key dissonance
timpani clash
silent radioactivity light the path

noiseless gray measure
blasts out doses in 32 performances
without missing a beat
this is no backstreet John Philip Sousa
pores and tissues play their part
invisible, audible, present

it's big band warfare
trombone thrombosis
drumming down deep in molecular time
contrapuntal light field
sparks rhythmically
fractionated in 4:4 time
to drown out malignancy
and cure before finale

let the heat of the music
be remedy,
the full throttle of its vibration
faster than the speed of cancer.

Waiting Room

My crimson neck heralds my arrival
I pretend I am to be suited for war
with a mask that hangs on the wall
it bears my name but needs no identity
all the jousters' masks resemble the faces
sitting outside the radiation room
outlines still, robotic

we wait for the flying saucer
to move inquiringly about our heads
shooting external-beam rays
into head, neck and nodes
waiting doesn't cease
beyond the waiting room

after daily treatment
paragraphs are spoken
in comrades' eyes
one emerges in tears but
no words are exchanged
soothing is transmitted in glances
like old trees in the night woods
intertwining their branches

get up, walk around a corner
find sunlight reaching
across impeccable windows
count the squares on the carpet
notice the knife-shaped sun streak on the
sidewalk below. No need to protect your eyes,
waiting temporarily eclipsed by blinding

pacing induces several trips
to the sterile bathroom
to pump the foam soap
watch the sink bubble up to the brim
then swirl into the drain
imagine how pain goes down

at the final session
no one sits
expectantly waiting
when I ring the Victory bell
radiating the glow of
a thousand southern suns
waiting doesn't cease
beyond the waiting room.

Rx

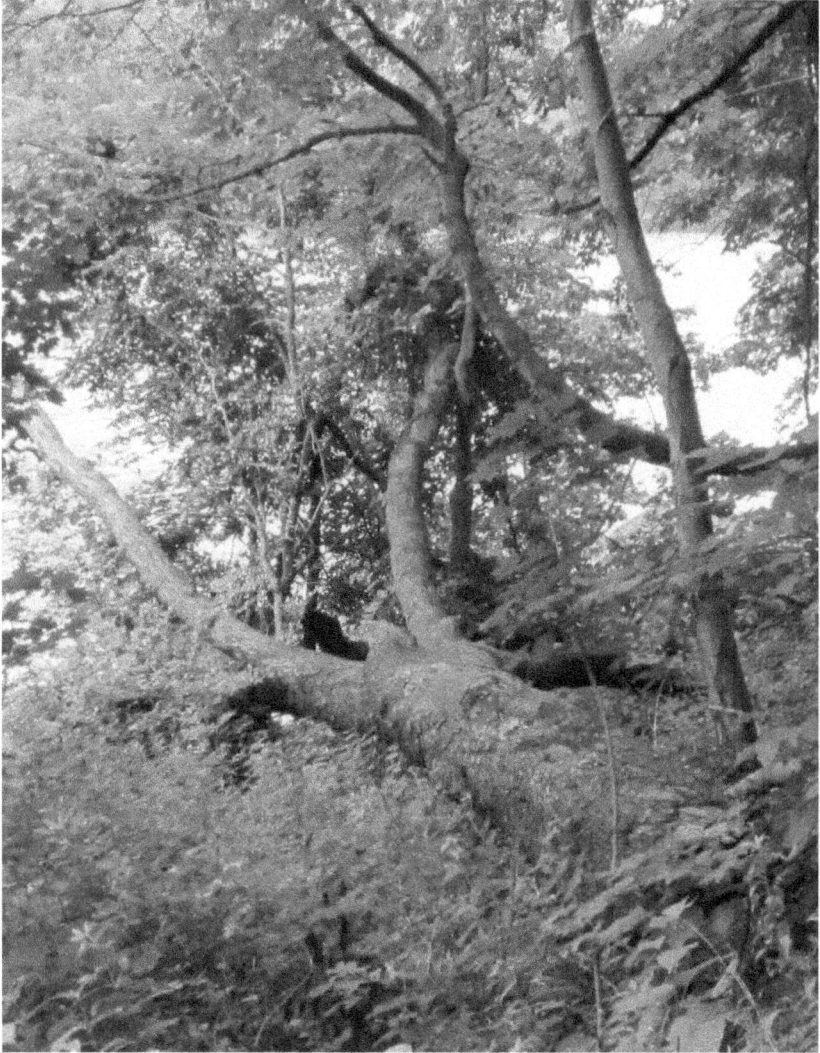

Rejuvenation Among the Dying

There is a moment
when you awaken in the dark
you don't know where you are
that single instance of wellness
clock hands turned back
mistake never made
forgiven or never spoken

G-Floor is very quiet this night
every night, it turns out
I lie unknowing
among the terminally ill

tentative euphoria
and immeasurable guilt
waste my poisoned cells
I listen to the verdict
for twelve patients
that I alone will live

reluctant to push the button
that will relieve my night discomfort
of singed neck and head
the alternative is to turn
to morphine illusions of
psychedelic muted colors
human feet dancing beneath terra cotta pots

merging souls to Kama Sutra drumbeats
this world is not pleasant here
eyes closed, mind open

wellness between post-REM
and rude awakening
has a different light
at the end of its tunnel
an 85-90% chance my sun
will have multiple risings
bedside flowers will pass
but many more bouquets
will ring my front doorbell
I resemble a Hiroshima victim
irradiated head, neck and body
will move slightly scarred
through the unscathed
for an unspecified tomorrow

rooms joined in a circle
fanning out from the nurse station
a carousel, a bicycle
my room the uneven spoke
the cog in the wheel
a spider, a sun
twelve hours a day
twelve months a year
twelve signs of the zodiac

laughter breaks through the pin-drop halls
nobody seems to wait here killing time
all our minutes tick and tock
am I making mine count too?

Nurse enters briefly to refresh,
remove the morning evidence
of existing with cancer
How much did you eat?
she refers to a removed waffle plate
baked into the shape of Texas
I attempt to describe the absence of food
Houston, Austin and Dallas, I answer
she smiles and says: *good*

subdued quiet
a single moment of wellbeing
we are part of the whole
a reluctant sun outside
is rising in my east
while it is setting
for these weary eleven jurors

this misjudgment is harsh
as each closes eyes
for the night
for keeps.

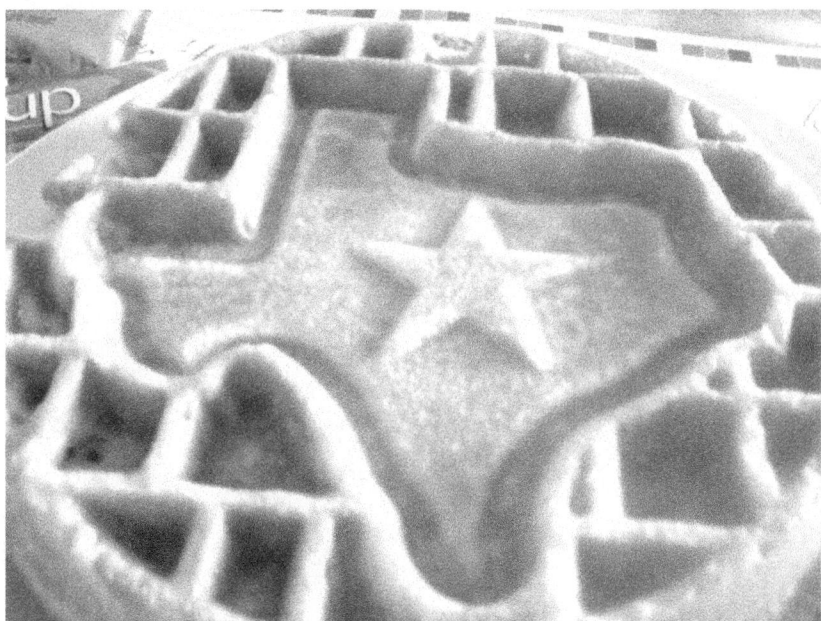

Recovery

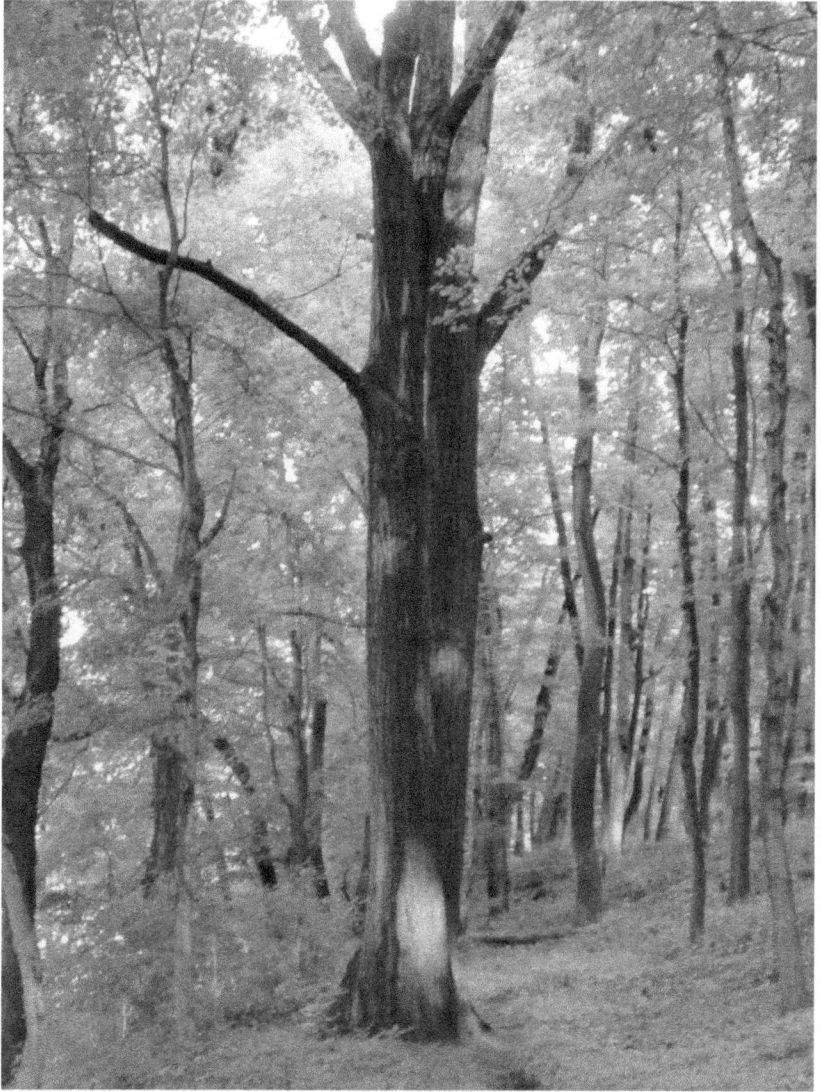

Recovery on Lopez Island

The ferry ride from Anacortes
to Lopez is sublime
each whitecap resembles a seal
my sister sits by me on the sunny side
she inspects the novel I'm holding
and asks to borrow it; it's not mine
I show her the inscription
she notices a large spider on the
inside cover, shrieks
the book flies across the ferry
we laugh at her fear

recovery is fear without the edge
it lingers at Ground Zero
with cryptic anticipation
I endure *how are you*
you look great, I would never know
you're all healed, right?
I nod and feel their relief
a war officially declared over
casualties are unloaded in flag-draped coffins
nothing is clean

later we hike on a narrow
wood-chipped path through lush forestation
I hear the cries of roots underfoot
scores of naturalists plod through with bodies

and faces sacrificed to the Pacific sun
wearing protective gear to the extreme
I hopscotch on the path between
the knuckles of ancient trees

everything is in recovery
tide comes in after it recedes
water's smooth skin returns when a ferry passes
calmness breathes after a fit of arachnophobia
even tree roots adapt
from intruder footsteps

recovery is self-forgiveness
not only for the path not taken
lovers not loved
but joy dismissed
a last uneaten yellow banana
left on the counter to over-ripen
by the unselfish

on Lopez Island I sit for a long time
on jagged rocks pretending
I am a large blubbery seal
stretched across a pointed reef
carpeted with barnacles
nose to the water, fins skyward
not backward, just forward.

Après Recovery

In Diagnostic Testing
a woman murmurs
every day is a day
you're not going to have again
post-treatment dessert course
medic butlers in blue
mixed among weightless patients
in pale blankets and cautious eyes
blinking above face masks
certainty of après-cure
offered under an oven
of camera, lights, devices
one after-dinner serving, s'il vous plait
intravenous contrast
comparative studies
of what you looked like
before and after malignant tumors
giant microscope peers within
hungry soul poised to be of use
people in different phases
of the meal seated quietly
focusing on the next repast
a menu above a door
Cancer Changes Things
ubiquitous stuffed animal
stretched across a child's knees
as she waits for her name
to be called.

Haiku

Molecular storm
science defies hurricane
disease exiting

Bleak view of open plains
post woodland excavation
moss grows on felled limbs

Time not essential
transformation alters path
breathe honeysuckle

Assimilation

No longer breathing diagnosis
stark raving pain in the distance,
mixing with the ill
is becoming a foreign country

such as dim memories of trips
when Sedona vortex
enabled steep mountain climb
or heart pounding
on deserted Venice
river backstreets
of thieves and putrid waters

regime of enemy overthrown
DNA thwarted
whether luck
or hope
or perceived intervention
body healed by poison and fire
reversal of misfortune

final movement
assimilation among the resilient.

Side Effects

The throat is useful for silence

how many times do we need to recuperate
from swallowing our pride or words
Ensure or large pills that are trapped
on the railroad crossing
of the pharyngeal contraction

the time to nap nears when my wind-up
toy body is on its last rotation
it feels so good to give in

but first I wrap my lymph-obstructed
neck like an Egyptian
then climb into a sweet bedstead
and inhale the aroma of 375-threadcount
I lie threadbare and anxious
for a different tomorrow
which doesn't come from sleep

the throat wants to leave
the hot coals of radiation aftermath
and fantasizes climbing
into the mouth of an auctioneer
or a mute.

Elegy

I never thought I'd mourn a lymph node
tenants unannounced
swept my passages
removed liquid waste

a tornado takes something with it
when it cleans house
just indentation remains

the song of tall trees
is hushed;
either wind is missing
or it's the trees themselves
lost in the meddling
of an interloper
who at heart wants to heal me

I was told before anesthetic sleep
some of my body parts
would be evacuated for a time
like levee-break victims swimming
searching for home

if I die
I want to recognize
myself when I return
a root, a curl
smooth, untroubled skin

but I am missing you
I look for you
in necks of passersby
but you're not coming back
any of you, *are* you?

Omen

The thirty minutes after biopsy
is nothing less than a lifetime

cry, pray, watch an unmoving clock
see an hour pass in a minute

life becomes suddenly uncluttered
two women exit Diagnostic Testing

neither greeting the other
terror mingles from eyes to eyes.

Remembering on a particular day
in my coming-of-age neighborhood

skies lacked clarity as they wrapped
the earth in sour discontent

birds frenetically traded places
across nervous trees

a foretelling only known to insects
and pre-tsunami elephants
heading for stable ground

the road became taffy
stretching and thinning
wind pulled and heaved

that day, arrival home after school
as if ominous breath followed me

gave way to a thud on the floor above
upstairs my sister's parakeet lay still

at cage bottom, her own
homecoming imminent.

Ultrasounds and scans happen with regularity
without warning of thunder or troubled sky

the pendulum of positive-negative
swings madly

like a bird's recently abandoned perch
prognosis: g o o d.

Now, predict the shelf life
of a sigh of relief.

Labyrinth

An odyssey
doesn't come with
an instruction manual

body begins as a small person
stretching with growth
receding in old age
mutating, regenerating

k e e p   m o v i n g

make your pilgrimage fearlessly
no matter what course
cells may take

if there is a way in
there is a way out

walk the continuum
follow its metastasis

taste the unfolding
narrative.

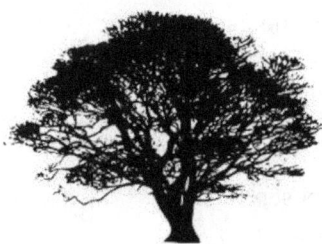

Catch of the Day

First lesson in fly fishing:
Bend the barb down

it protects the fish
and it's easy to release
but an ultra-light drag line
will cause a struggle
before it is revived
and the fish fights longer
it's not so easy to reel it in
as with a heavy line
this tires out the fish.

More lessons:
Set the drag on the reel

tighten or loosen the line
the lighter the drag,
you won't snap the line

when you re-introduce a fish
move water over the gills
so it can catch its breath
it recovers, then you let it go.

The floating period
before recovery -
the tether that binds us
often saves us

the swim upstream
is a delicate journey

a fish released
the triumph after battle.

Notes

Chapter Headings

Fx, Dx, Tx, Rx are common references used in notes by the American medical community regarding patients, denoting Fracture, Diagnosis, Treatment, Prescription. Other standard abbreviations include Sx (Symptoms) and Hx (History).

"Bomb Shelter"

Refers to American school children who were taught to "duck and cover." In case of nuclear attack they were herded into school hallways and basements for bomb drills after concern over Russia's launch of Sputnik I and the Cuban Missile Crisis.

"Isotopes"

Some isotopes are radioactive and are described as radioisotopes. The energy given off by radioisotopes can be effectively used to zap diseased cells. When delivered straight to cancer cells, healthy tissues are spared while cancer cells may be eliminated.

"Tenth Floor"

This poem, and others in this collection, refers to treatment received at MD Anderson Cancer Center. A multidisciplinary approach to treatment was pioneered at MD Anderson which utilizes teams of experts across disciplines to collaborate on a treatment plan. It is the only NCI–designated comprehensive cancer facility with its own Emergency Center.

"66 Gy Led the Big Parade"

The amount of radiation is measured in gray (Gy) and varies depending on the type and stage of cancer being treated. The gray was named after the British physicist Louis Harold Gray, a pioneer in the field of measurement of radium radiation and X-rays and their effects on living tissue. For curative cases, the typical dose for a solid epithelial tumor ranges from 60 to 80 Gy, while lymphomas are treated with 20 to 40 Gy. The poem title is based on the song, "76 Trombones" from *The Music Man*.

"Haiku"

Haiku is a very short form of Japanese poetry typically characterized by 17 syllables in three phrases of 5, 7 and 5. Nature and the passing of time are often thematic elements. The earliest haiku poets are documented as living during the 17th century in Japan. Previously called *hokku*, haiku was given its current name by the Japanese writer, Masoka Shiki at the end of the 19th century.

"Labyrinth"

Labyrinths are thought of as symbolic forms of pilgrimage. Labyrinths substituted for travel to holy sites and lands. Their spiritual aspect has experienced a resurgence. It is felt that walking among the turns may lead to transformative enlightenment.

i thank You God for most this amazing
day:for the leaping greenly spirits of trees

— e. e. cummings

About the Author

Susan Kerschner's poems have appeared in *Arts Connection*, *BardFest 2000 Anthology*, *Shirazad*, *Circle Magazine*, small press periodicals including *River Poets* (Lily Press), *The River* of Bucks County, Pa. and online literary magazines. In 2002, she was selected to participate in the *Poets & Painters* exhibit at the *Berks Arts Council Gallery at the Reading Pagoda*, Reading, Pa. One of the original members of *Berks Bards* in Southeastern Pennsylvania in 1995, the author also won awards at the *Summit Arts Competition*, Schuylkill County, Pa. in 1997 and 1998. She is a judge in the annual *Young Poets* competition in Berks County, Pa. schools, grades K-12. A Spoken Word CD project is scheduled to be released entitled *Forest of You*, a collection of her poetry with acoustic music accompaniment.

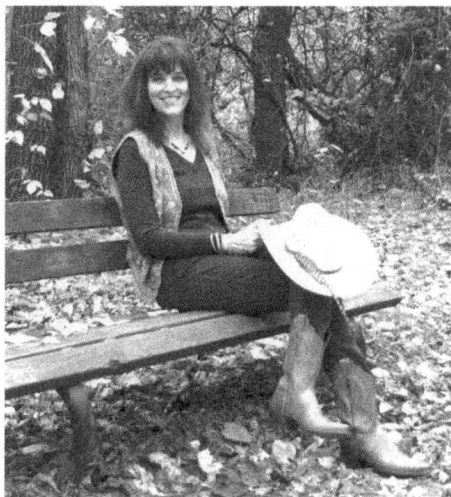

www.ingramcontent.com/pod-product-compliance
Lightning Source LLC
Chambersburg PA
CBHW021838020426
42334CB00014B/681